Low Fat Cookbook

A Low Fat Diet with Gluten Free Recipes

Duane Hill

Table of Contents

LOW FAT COOKBOOK INTRODUCTION 1

SECTION 1: GLUTEN FREE COOKBOOK 6

What is Gluten? 7
Advantages of Going Gluten Free 8
Gluten Free Cooking 9
What Makes Gluten Free a Good Choice? 11
Making Gluten-Free Work for You 11
Gluten Intolerance and Allergies 13
What Are You Giving Up? 14

MAIN DISH GLUTEN FREE RECIPES. 16

Lamb with Yams and Apples 16
Cheesy Mexican Chicken 19
Broiled Steak Salad 21
Hearty Steak and Cheese Soup 23
Beef and Broccoli 25
Curried Chicken and Mango Summer Salad 28

HEALTH CHALLENGES IN OUR WORLD 30

SIDE DISHES AND VEGETABLES 31

Winter Squash in Brown Butter and Parsley 32
Chinese Green Beans 34
High Energy Breakfast Smoothie 36
Heart Healthy Spinach Side Salad 37
Creamy Broccoli and Cauliflower Salad 40
Hearty Summer Salad 42

APPETIZERS AND SNACKS 45

Garlic and Parmesan Chicken Wings 46
Hot and Spicy Chicken Wings 48

TIPS ON "SNACKABLE" TREATS 49

GLUTEN FREE CONSERVES AND RELISHES 51
Raw Salsa 52
Home Made Spicy Salsa 52
Cranberry Conserve 54

GLUTEN FREE DESSERTS - YES, THEY CAN BE HEALTHY 56
Hot Chocolate Pudding 57
FAST and Easy Gluten Free Rice Pudding 59
Chocolate Fondue Dessert 61
Dark Chocolate Fondue 61
Gluten Free Chocolate Cake 63
Baked Apples 65
Coffee Chocolate Mousse 67

GLUTEN FREE TIPS FOR FUN KID FOODS 69
Gluten Free Breakfast Idea 69
Gluten Free Chocolate Chip Cookies 71

CROCK POT COOKERY AND GLUTEN FREE? 73
Restaurant Foods on a Gluten Free Diet 76

TIPS ON LIVING GLUTEN FREE: 78

REFERENCES AND CREDITS 81

SECTION 2: GLUTEN FREE VEGAN 84

GLUTEN 86
Celiac Disease 86

VEGAN LIFESTYLE AND DIET 89
History 89

Philosophy..89

GLUTEN FREE VEGAN ALTERNATIVE INGREDIENTS . 91
Eggs...91
Flour..92
Butter..94
Milk Substitutes 95
Vegan Pasta...96
Gluten Free Vegan Pie Crust..97

GLUTEN FREE VEGAN RECIPES...............................99

SNACKS 99
Onion Rings 99
Sweet Potato Fries...101
Peanut Butter Apple (quick snack).......................................102

MAIN DISHES...103
Vegetables and Rice...103
Chickpea Salad..105
Pasta Marinara...106
Simple Mexican Stew...108
Simple Spanish Rice 109
Vegetable Pot Pie 111

SIDE DISHES...113
Potato Rice Balls..113
Vegan Baked Potato...114
Chestnut Rissoles 116
Polenta and Corn...117

DESSERTS 119
Zucchini Banana Spice Cake...119
Creamy Apple Tapioca 121
Strawberries in Cherry Syrup...122
Banana Nut Bread 123
Vegan Gluten Free Chocolate Chip Cookies 125

SOUPS 127

Gluten Free Vegan Tomato Soup 127

Hearty Mexican Soup 129

Potato, Squash and Apple Soup 130

French Cabbage Soup 131

RAW FOODS, SEASONAL FAVORITES AND DRINKS.132

Pineapple Banana Drink 132

Bacon- Sort Of! 133

"Eggnog" 134

Vegan Cocoa 135

Holiday Favorite Pumpkin Pie 136

GLUTEN FREE VEGAN STAPLES FOR THE PANTRY .137

HEALTH CONCERNS OF A VEGAN GLUTEN FREE DIET 139

Vitamin B-12 139

Iron 140

Omega-3 Fatty Acids 141

Calcium 141

Gluten Free Concerns 142

GLUTEN FREE VEGAN CONCLUSION 144

VEGAN FAQ'S 145

Is a vegan diet healthy? 145

How difficult is it to go vegan? 145

Is a vegan diet expensive? 145

GLUTEN FREE FAQ'S 147

What foods can I eat? 147

Why are oats such a big deal? 147

Is celiac disease really that bad? 147

GLUTEN FREE VEGAN -- IN SUMMARY 150

Low Fat Cookbook Introduction

These days all you have to do is step outside if you want to be bombarded by a number of ads showing you the benefits of dieting. On the other end of the spectrum however, you will also see advertisements encouraging you to eat unhealthy foods. The commercials on television certainly do not hint at the fact that some are deadly, and to be perfectly honest, many fast food companies do not really pay attention to food related regulations. While the occasional burger might taste good, you would probably be better off making it at home. This book covers a number of different fast food alternatives, particularly the gluten free diet. This is likely something you have heard of before – gluten free that is. What is it? Why does it work? Why should you consider it?

There are a few reasons that people will choose to go the gluten free route, but before we start, what is gluten? Gluten is often found in wheat products, and it can actually be pretty harmful to the body. In addition to that it might actually increase your cravings for processed foods. When the body gets used to something, it does not like to give it up. If you can however get your body hooked on gluten free foods, you might find that it is easier to take the right path.

The human body is not capable of fully digesting wheat, and the undigested parts will actually begin to ferment within the body. This forms gas, similar to the reaction to milk by those who are lactose intolerant. In addition to that, the body's insulin levels can rise, which causes inflammation at the cellular level. Refined wheat does not have much in the way of nutritional value, meaning you are not missing much by cutting out of your diet. As one of the top eight allergens, it is no surprise that millions of people have a gluten sensitivity without even realizing it. It has been estimated that 1 in 100 people have celiac disease, though this is not certain, as most people have no idea. After all, there are bigger medical problems to worry about!

When you are heading to the grocery store with the intention of purchasing gluten free foods, you need to plan ahead, and know exactly what you are going to buy. You should make a list on either paper, or your tablet if you happen to have one. If you know what you are going to buy, you don't have to waste time checking ingredients, and you do not have to worry about impulse purchases. Through this system you will save both your health AND your money!

When you are buying gluten free, you should take into account that there are two different types of gluten free foods. One type is naturally gluten free, and the others are specialty items made by companies. You can buy either one, but make sure that you buy what tastes good to YOU. The last thing you want to do is choose a meal that doesn't taste good! The idea here is to replace your meals with something that alleviates your cravings for the more unhealthy foods, and you cannot do that if it doesn't taste good.

You can do your shopping for gluten free food at the grocery store, but if you want a bit more variety, it might be a good idea to visit ethnic and farmer's markets. As a last ditch effort, you might use the internet as gluten free ingredients can be sent directly to your door if you wish.

When you are partaking of the gluten free diet you will want to avoid certain foods. We will not list all of them, but they can include:

Beer
Cornbread
Cereal

Bread

Croutons

Liquorice

Marinades

Pasta

Gravy

Soy Sauce

Stuffing

While this might cut out 90% of your weekly diet, you will be pleased to find that there is a substitute for nearly everything you love. No, a substitute might not be 'good enough', but that doesn't mean you should dismiss it entirely. Taking on a diet like this will give you the relief your body really needs for a few reasons. You will feel better initially, and before you know it you will be considerably healthier. The toughest part of starting a diet of course is sticking to it, and if you can just set a goal for yourself, you can try to meet that goal, and reward yourself for doing so.

One of the most important parts of dieting however is to keep a record of your success. If it appears that you are not making any headway, you might become discouraged and give up. The thing to remember however, is that you WILL have some measure of success, and with that being the case, you need to record it. As you see yourself improve you will be more and more motivated to move on, ultimately becoming the person you truly want to be. It might sound far fetched, but there are many success stories, and within the pages of this e-book, you will find the solution to a great number of your problems. Whether you're stressed, depressed, or generally unhappy with your life, you will find that the right diet and a fair amount of exercise can take you to the finish line. After all, you have nothing to lose by giving it a try, right?

Section 1: Gluten Free Cookbook

Gluten Free diets are typically entered into by necessity, not by chance. That doesn't mean, however, that there are no real benefits to making the choice to go gluten free. In fact, for those who are considering a diet that may help to lower their cholesterol and make other positive, long-term health changes, going gluten free has some potential health benefits that may not have been considered.

Going gluten free has become a fairly popular new trend. You might even consider it to be one of those diet "fads" that hit the magazine and book shelves every few years. The difference is that most fads are not healthy and really don't help a great deal. This fad--which is not really a fad--is being seen to increase the energy and to improve the overall good health of many people who use it.

Celebrities such as Gwyneth Paltrow and Chelsea Clinton are finding that gluten free works for them, and it can work for you too. It's quite likely that you're seeing more and more gluten free products hitting the supermarket shelves recently. For those who have no food allergies and aren't concerned with gluten in their diet, going gluten free is something you probably haven't explored very carefully. The reason for the growing number of gluten free foods is that many people have explored gluten free and found that even if they don't' have to utilize the diet, it's much healthier--quite like the paleo diets which are so popular.

What is Gluten?

Gluten is a kind of protein that is part of grains and cereal products such as wheat. It tends To make bread and foods elastic, or chewy tasting. It keeps food from being "sticky." Gluten is found in flour products of wheat, but more, it is also found in other grains.

There are such a wide range of people who have a problem with gluten that it is considered to be one of the big 8 which are mandated to be listed on food packaging. If you have a gluten intolerance or allergy, going gluten free for you isn't a choice, it's a necessity and you need To make sure that you don't accidentally take in gluten in some form by mistake.

Become an expert at reading the packaging and finding

out precisely what is in the product and not just that, what it has come into contact with so that you know your products are gluten free.

People who have certain food allergies or disease processes such as Celiac disease may not be able to tolerate even a tiny amount of gluten in their diet. One of the most common questions to be found among those who are newly diagnosed with Celiac is what they can and cannot eat. Take that a step further and realize that not only edible products have gluten, but many inedible ones do as well. Be very careful to wash your hands after using some soaps, lotions and even pet foods as these have nominal amounts of gluten in them which could be transferred to your food if you don't wash carefully after using them.

Advantages of Going Gluten Free

Doctors and naturalists have taken a good look at gluten free diets recently and found that gluten free can help to improve the overall good health of even those who are not suffering from a gluten allergy.

It can help to improve your serum cholesterol level, may also promote better digestion, and might even increase your energy, particularly if you may be suffering from a gluten allergy or intolerance. The reason for this is not that gluten itself is particularly unhealthy. Many of the foods which are made from gluten or with gluten incorporated into them tend to be less healthy than those which do not contain it.

Gluten Free Cooking

Gluten free foods impose some big challenges. It makes it hard to enjoy foods that you may have eaten your entire life, but with a little work, you can make those recipes your own and in many cases, you'll be surprised at what foods are out there are naturally gluten free.

For example, a vanilla milkshake made with all natural ice cream is normally gluten free. Fresh strawberries, spinach, fruits of nearly all types and vegetables are gluten free naturally.

Even many of your favorite snack foods will be gluten free. Potato chips and most corn chips which are fried or baked in corn oil or soybean oil are gluten free. Check the packaging, but most are baked or fried using heart healthy methods and so are gluten free without any help from you. While these are not the ideal snacks, they are able to be eaten in moderation.

While it may be moderately frustrating at first trying to replace things like cake flour and find ways To make pasta and cookies, the more you look at gluten free meals, the more you'll find that you can create nearly any recipe that you like with gluten free foods and emulate most any recipe that you'll find with common sense and a bit of skill in substitution.

Take a look your new diet and approach it with the attitude of exploring new things, a challenge rather than a chore and you'll find that in no time, you and your family have really conquered the world of gluten free cooking. You may even find that you enjoy cooking more and that eating is more fun, better tasting, and healthier by far than those which incorporate the very sticky gluten filled processed foods that you were accustomed to.

Which Foods Would Be Eliminated in a Gluten Free Diet?

In many cases, the foods which are not healthy for you anyway, particularly processed foods would be missing from your diet. Foods such as white bread, white crackers and other processed wheat products are going to be eliminated from your diet. Noodles of many types are foods which won't be allowed to be eaten, but they can be replaced with rice noodles and other forms of pasta which are healthy and tasty.

The problem is that many people like the taste of these foods, and don't consider the many unhealthy components that are part of them. Foods which are processed such as supermarket breads and pastries contain not just gluten, but unhealthy fats, many preservatives, and other chemicals that are higher in disease promoting ingredients.

What Makes Gluten Free a Good Choice?

Studies show that eating a low gluten or gluten free diet can lower your risk of some disease processes such as heart disease, certain types of cancer, type 2 diabetes, and many other long term health conditions. Your diet would be richer in fruits and vegetables and would quite likely contain many more foods that offer positive health benefits and a higher level of vitamins, phytonutrients, and antioxidants.

Making Gluten-Free Work for You

Every year more and more people are diagnosed with celiac disease. They are required to eat a gluten free diet. You perhaps are not required to go gluten free, but the health benefits of doing so are nothing short of amazing. Even if you do not have celiac disease or an allergy to gluten which compels you to avoid oats, wheat, rye and malt, if you follow the gluten free diet even loosely, you may find that you feel better, that your skin is much clearer, and that you may have a lower incidence of heartburn, fatigue, and cramping.

The poor vitamin absorption that takes place in Celiac disease can make the person who suffers from this disease feel very unwell, have side effects of loose stool and even depression. It is imperative to stay within the dietary restrictions which have been given to you and to understand why you have those restrictions.

Basing your diet on a gluten free approach may be a good idea, but for the Celiac sufferer, it's something that is non-optional. The very strict limitations that apply to the celiac sufferer would not apply to those who are making a choice to go gluten-free, but sticking as closely as you can to the gluten-free approach will improve your health by removing most of the high fats and fried foods that we should quite likely be avoiding anyway. It can be a genuinely healthy way to eat, improving your serum cholesterol and your energy. It's not necessary to be as strict with yourself, such as avoiding malt flavors, when you are not genuinely restricted, but staying close to the diet so far as main meal ingredients will be beneficial for your entire family.

Gluten Intolerance and Allergies

Today for whatever reason, many people are actively allergic to gluten, to wheat and to other components of wheat. The numbers of these people grow continuously every year. It is particularly difficult in the case of children to limit gluten in the diet. If their allergic reaction is bad enough, the reaction can be devastating and foods which have gluten must be completely eliminated. Using rice noodles and gluten free foods is an imperative, not a choice. In addition, some diseases exist which require that people who suffer from them do not have gluten of any type as part of their diet. This means that not only wheat, but other foods which contain gluten must be eliminated from the diet.

Celiac is a serious illness with real consequences if the sufferer does not eliminate gluten. Keep in mind that making the choice to go gluten free means that you can be a little more lenient with yourself. You may eat foods such as soy sauce and other things that are not available to the sufferer of celiac or gluten intolerance. To that end, our book contains only recipes that are strictly and completely gluten free in order to be useful to the user who has chosen to go gluten free, as well as to the celiac client, who has a need to follow a strict gluten free method of eating.

What Are You Giving Up?

One of the first comments that people make when considering a gluten free diet is that they won't be able to enjoy desserts and other things that they are accustomed to and simply want on an occasional basis. The fact is that some things will be off limits, specifically processed pastries and that type of foods. That doesn't mean that there is nothing to replace it.

Eliminating gluten from your diet does not mean sacrificing taste. In fact, quite the opposite. Many of the things that you eat on a gluten free diet will be sweet treats that you make yourself. They won't incorporate high fat and gluten, of course, but they will incorporate fresh fruits, even cocoa in some cases, so you won't lose your chocolate or some of the other foods that you love. They can be eaten sparingly and when created with the correct ingredients don't add gluten or even a high amount of empty calories to your meals.

Gluten Free foods don't have to be lacking in taste or fiber. Here are some wonderful examples of what can be done with gluten free cooking, listed for you in sections.

Main Dish Gluten Free Recipes.

Main dish recipes are one of the most difficult to accomplish without any gluten but with a little imagination and creativity, you can come up with some wonderful meals that are gluten free and have incredible taste and appeal. Some perfect examples of gluten free main dish recipes include these, which are all created for the person who really has to have no gluten at all incorporated into their diet.

Lamb with Yams and Apples

This is completely gluten free and offers great taste as well as ample nutrition. The pairing of apples and yams offers a little sweetness to the pork as well as keeping it moist.

You will need:

- 1/4 cup dark brown sugar
- 5 tablespoons butter, melted
- 1 tsp vinegar
- 1 tsp salt
- 1/2 tsp granulated garlic

- 2 apples, cored and sliced
- 2 sweet potatoes, peeled and sliced
- 2 chops, preferably the tenderloin style

To make:

Preheat oven to 400 degrees Fahrenheit.

Mix the sugar, the butter the vinegar and the spices.

Keep about a tablespoon of the butter mix and set it aside.

Add the apple and sweet potato to your brown sugar mix and coat them.

Place the apples and potatoes in a roasting pan and cover with foil. Bake for twenty minutes.

Meanwhile lightly brown the lamb in the remaining butter mix.

Remove the potato and apple mixture from the oven and add the lamb over the top of the mix.

Replace the dish in the oven and bake it for approximately 40 minutes until a meat thermometer shows that the lamb is cooked.

Cheesy Mexican Chicken

Cheesy chicken becomes an instant favorite when you create it combined with cheese. Low in fat and high in nutrients, chicken is a favorite food for about half the world. This has a bit of a bite to it, with the chili peppers and tomato added

You will need:

- 2 tablespoon of olive oil
- 1 can diced tomatoes
- 1/2 teaspoon sea salt
- fresh ground pepper
- 1/2 cup finely chopped green onion
- 1 chopped clove of garlic
- 1 tsp chopped fresh cilantro
- 1 can diced green chilies
- 1 can black beans
- 1/3 cup Colby jack cheese
- 2 cups cooked white rice

To make:

Chop the chicken into cubes and brown in the olive oil, sprinkling with the sea salt and pepper.

Add the remaining ingredients, excluding the cheese.

Allow to cook on the stove top on low heat for approximately 40 minutes, until chicken is thoroughly cooked and tender.

Serve over white rice, topped with shredded Colby jack cheese.

Broiled Steak Salad

Broiled steak offers a chance for a great deal of the fat from the meat to leak into the broiler tray below, while not using the grilling that has been shown to cause some health considerations. Broiling meat and adding it to the wide array of greens and fresh vegetables ends up with a healthy and delicious meal that is gluten free and oh-so delicious.

You will need:

- 4 tablespoons of olive oil
- 6 teaspoons of apple cider vinegar
- 1 teaspoon fresh cilantro, chopped
- 2 tablespoons of fresh parsley, finely chopped
- 1 bell pepper sliced in strips
- 3 finely chopped green onions
- 1 clove garlic, minced
- 2 Roma or other meaty tomato, diced
- salt and pepper to taste.
- 2 cups romaine lettuce
- 2 cups iceberg lettuce
- 2 cups baby spinach
- 1/2 cup raw mushrooms
- 1/4 cup part skim mozzarella cheese
- 2 sirloin or Delmonico steaks

To make:

Take one quarter of the garlic, and rub steaks.

Salt and pepper steaks to taste, and place below the broiler.

Allow steaks to broil turning once until cooked to your taste.

Tear greens, mix and set aside.

Combine remaining ingredients and set aside.

Remove steaks from the broiler and cut into strips about half an inch wide

Place greens into salad plates and top with strips of the steak.

Sprinkle with grated mozzarella

Drizzle the vegetable dressing over the steak and the salad greens till coated. Serve warm.

Hearty Steak and Cheese Soup

Steak soup is a hearty way to end the day and perfect for those cooler autumn or winter days. If you're ready for a warm ending to the day, you can add the veggies and meats to your crock pot and leave on low heat for about 6 hours and your soup will be ready for you when you arrive home after work.

Fresh raw vegetables are the best that you can get and will give your soup a wonderful flavor, but in the event that your raw veggies are off season, frozen vegetables will work nearly as well and most of the time does not cause the nutrients to erode. If you're really hungry, consider adding some canned or dried beans to your soup To make it a bit more hearty and rib-sticking.

You will need:

- 2 lbs. stew meat or diced steak
- 2 quart cans of tomato juice
- 2 cups beef broth
- 1/4 cup frozen corn
- 1/3 cup chopped green onion
- 1/3 cup chopped celery hearts
- 1 cup halved baby carrots
- 1 cup diced potatoes

- 1 cup tomatoes diced
- 1 cup whole green beans-raw
- 2 tsp. Sea salt
- freshly ground black pepper
- 1 clove garlic-finely chopped
- 1/2 cup chopped green pepper
- 1 cup shredded cheddar or Colby Jack cheese to top the soup.

To make:

Into 1 qt. of water put beef and boil for 1 hour on medium heat.

For a hearty, substantial soup, cut up the meat in small pieces and add salt and pepper to taste.

Add tomatoes, tomato juice, onions and celery. Also add other vegetables, such as diced potatoes, carrots, string beans, corn, peas, cabbage or chopped peppers.

Boil until all vegetables are tender.

Serve topped with shredded cheddar and then broil it for just a moment To make the cheese bubbly.

Beef and Broccoli

One of the favorite Chinese foods which can be created is the beef and broccoli that we all eat on our forays out to the Chinese restaurant. This recipe can be made gluten free and also a bit healthier by the removal of a few things and the addition of another set. Keeping your foods heart healthy as well as gluten free means not using some of the traditional Chinese food inclusions such as monosodium glutamate, but in many cases, with the right spices, you're not even going to miss it.

It typically comes as a surprise to people that soy sauce is not gluten free traditionally. Soy sauce does tend to have wheat in it, but you can get around that with several brands of soy sauce that are fermented naturally and do not include gluten. The gluten free soy sauce has the same great taste that you'd come to expect. While we did name a brand that we know to be gluten free, bear in mind that there are others and this is simply a guideline.

You will need:

1 pound lean beef, sliced thinly into bite-sized pieces.

Marinade for Beef:

- 1 egg
- 1/3 tsp salt
- 1 Tbsp stock
- 1 Tbsp cornstarch (corn flour)
- 2 Tbsp water

Remaining ingredients:

- 1 1/2 Tbsp sunflower oil
- 1 16 ounce bag of broccoli,
- 1 cup sunflower oil
- 2 Tbsp Kikkoman Gluten-Free Soy Sauce
- 1 Tbsp sugar
- a few drops of sesame oil
- 2 cloves garlic, crushed
- 1/2 cup chicken broth
- 2 Tbsp cornstarch

To make:

Slice your beef into tiny pieces and add it to the marinade. Marinate the beef for at least half hour before adding the 1 1/2 tablespoons of oil to beef, mixing it all in and marinating your beef for another half hour.

While the beef is getting ready in the marinade, you'll be using that time to prepare the vegetables.

Heat a wok or a heavy pot and add 1 cup of oil. Stir fry the beef and remove it, setting it aside on another plate. Drain the oil and wipe it clean of oil. Add one half cup of water to your pot and bring it to a boil, adding the broccoli to it. Cover and cook the broccoli after coming to a boil for about 5 minutes. Drain and remove the broccoli.

Heat the pan or wok with about 2 tablespoons of oil. Add the garlic and fry lightly. Add the veggies, the beef and mix them thoroughly. In the center of the pan, make a well of sorts and add all of the ingredients for the sauce. Stir the cornstarch into a tablespoon of water and use this to thicken your broth. Mix the sauce together with the other ingredients and serve hot accompanied by rice if you like.

Curried Chicken and Mango Summer Salad

Not only gorgeous because of the color, it's light and easy to accomplish for a summer meal. The main things which require any cooking are the chicken which can easily be broiled or grilled, keeping the kitchen heat to a minimum. Adding the mango to the meal makes it colorful and pretty, as well as lowering the calories and adding some phytonutrients. The yogurt adds a good dose of probiotics to your meal and all in all, this is one of the more healthy summertime quick meals you're going to find.

You will need:

- 3/4 cup plain Greek yogurt
- Juice of one half lime
- 2 teaspoons clover honey
- 1 teaspoon curry
- 1/8 teaspoon sea salt
- 1/8 teaspoon freshly ground pepper
- 2 cups cooked broiled chicken, cut into bite sized pieces
- 1 cup mango peeled and cubed
- About 10 leaves of Romaine lettuce

To make the salad:

Combine the first six ingredients in the list into a small bowl and stir it all really well.

Add the chicken and mango pieces and toss to coat.

On a salad plate, layer several leaves of crunchy Romaine.

Spoon the mango chicken mixture onto the top of the lettuce leaves and add a few pieces of chopped celery or cucumber for pretty and for crunch.

This delicious summer salad is also low in fat, low in calories and incorporates all of the health benefits that yogurt and mango have to offer.

Health Challenges in Our World

In the world today, some of the biggest challenges to our health include heart disease, stroke, Alzheimer's, cancer, and type 2 diabetes. Many of these things can be warded off if our diet becomes healthier and a little more natural. That means removing high fat foods, some of which are also high in gluten and replacing those foods with more natural foods such as fruits, vegetables and flour which is made of healthier ingredients. Whole grain foods are healthy in and of themselves, but once processed, contain additives which can be cancer-causing and high in fat.

Eliminating some of those foods can help To make a very positive change in your lifestyle and in your health. It may promote long term weight loss and change your life for the better. Adding more raw vegetables and even cooked or steamed will add further benefits to your long term good health.

Side Dishes and Vegetables

Vegetables are a very healthy part of your diet. So far as possible eating your vegetables raw is usually preferable in order to keep the nutrients sound. Many of the vitamins and minerals do not stay well during cooking or storage, with some being very unstable.

While there are exceptions to this rule, which will be named later, for the most part, keeping your vegetables raw will keep them more nutritious. Side dishes and salads are a very healthy part of your diet, combating some kinds of cancer as well as adding phytonutrients to your diet.

Winter Squash in Brown Butter and Parsley

Since this side-dish is prepared on the stovetop, it is especially nice for Thanksgiving and Christmas, when oven space always seems to be limited.

You will need:

- 1 ½ pounds winter squash, peeled, seeded, and cut into ½ inch cubes. (Acorn, or Butternut squash work well.)
- 4 Tbsp real butter
- 1 ½ Tbsp chopped, fresh parsley
- ¼ tsp salt
- ¼ tsp freshly ground black pepper
- 1 Tbsp brown sugar (optional)

To make:

Place butter in a large skillet over medium heat, stirring frequently with a whisk.

Once melted, the butter will foam a little, subside, milk solids will form and become a honey brown color. At this time the butter will have a strong nutty smell. (It take just a few seconds for your browned butter to burn, if this happens, you'll need to start over.)

Once the butter is browned, remove pan from heat and stir in fresh parsley.

Add cubed squash to pan, and turn to coat pieces evenly with butter, return to medium heat.

Allow the squash to cook on side until it is lightly browned. This usually takes a few minutes. Continue turning squash to evenly brown all sides.

Reduce heat to low, and cover. Let squash cook until fork tender, around ten minutes.

Add brown sugar, if desired, just before squash is done, and turn to distribute evenly.

Chinese Green Beans

We all love those delicious green beans that we get in the Chinese restaurant. The secret is the sesame oil in many cases, and you can make the same thing at home in a really short time. Using gluten free soy sauce, sesame oil and a few other ingredients, you can get all the taste that you want and absolutely none of the gluten that might be found in a restaurant offering. Try out this recipe for Chinese green beans and you may never have to find them at the restaurant again.

You will need:

- 1 pkg frozen green beans , one pound
- 1 tablespoon gluten free soy sauce
- 1 can gluten free chicken broth
- 1 bunch green onions, about six
- 2 cloves of garlic
- 1/4 tsp ground ginger
- 1 tsp sugar
- 1 tbsp sesame oil

To make:

In a 2-quart casserole dish, combine green beans and broth. Cover and microwave 4 minutes on high. Make sure that your dish is microwave safe and remove it with an oven mitt.

Meanwhile, chop the onion and mince garlic.

Into a small bowl, put the ginger, soy sauce and sugar.

Add scallion rings and garlic. Set aside. Remove green beans from microwave and uncover.

Pour sauce over beans and stir.

Add to the microwave again for approximately 3 minutes. Remove and ensure they are heated through. Stir in the sesame oil and serve immediately.

High Energy Breakfast Smoothie

Smoothies or breakfast shakes can be a very healthy way to start your day when you're in a hurry, as we all are in the morning. Getting a good dose of veggies and fruits in a way that everyone can enjoy means that you start your day with a good breakfast, avoid all the gluten, not to mention the sugar, that you're going to get from a normal wheat-laden breakfast and you'll have the energy you need to face the morning.

You will need:

- One medium sized banana
- 1 slice fresh pineapple
- 1/4 cup fresh blueberries
- 1/4 cup sliced strawberries
- 1 cup skim milk
- 1 tablespoon honey

To make:

Simply combine all ingredients and blend till smooth in a high speed blender.

Heart Healthy Spinach Side Salad

Salad is a very healthy side dish and is almost always gluten free, depending on the dressing that you get. This side salad features some very heart healthy additions and also greens which have been chosen for their nutritional phytonutrients. Additionally the presence of lycopene in the tomatoes as well as the Omega fatty acids which are found in the sunflower seeds offers you a real boost to your health.

You will need:
- 2 Roma tomatoes-quartered in wedges
- 2 cups Romaine lettuce
- 2 cups baby spinach leaves
- 2 cups iceberg lettuce
- 2 chopped green onions
- 1 cucumber, sliced in thin slices
- 2 tablespoons sunflower seeds

For the dressing:

- One quarter cup olive oil
- One quarter cup red wine vinegar
- 1 clove garlic, finely chopped

- 1 teaspoon cilantro chopped
- 1 teaspoon parsley , finely chopped

To make:

Combine the dressing ingredients and set aside. Allow to come to room temperature.

Quarter tomatoes.

Slice cucumbers carefully.

Break up the greens and alternate layers in two salad bowls.

Lay several tomato and cucumber slices arranged on top of the greens.

Shake the dressing gently to mix all ingredients and drizzle over the top of the greens and tomatoes.

Sprinkle liberally with sunflower seed.

Note. Tomatoes are very healthy; chock full of a nutrient called lycopene. The lycopene is a very good "anti-cancer" booster, but it requires either being cooked or a small amount of oil to be absorbed well. The olive oil in this salad dressing is actually a booster that will help the tomatoes to offer even more health benefits.

Creamy Broccoli and Cauliflower Salad

The tastes of raw broccoli and cauliflower were just made for summer time. This is an amazing taste treat and is also remarkably healthy. Cruciferous vegetables such as broccoli and cauliflower are not only heart healthy but may actually combat cancer and are high in vitamin A.

As quickly as this salad can be created and tasty as it is you may well find the perfect way to assure that your children will eat their veggies even in the summer time. The creamy taste of the salad comes from the slight amount of sour cream, but if you're concerned with calories, you'll get the same taste from a low fat sour cream. In order to create this salad, a small amount of milk can be used to thin the dressing slightly if needed.

You will need:

- One head of broccoli- chopped (not the stems)
- One head of cauliflower, cored and chopped
- 1/2 pound of precooked bacon,(about six slices) fried and chopped or crumbled
- 1/8 cup green onion very finely chopped
- 1/2 cup frozen green peas, thawed, but not cooked

- 1/2 cup grated cheddar cheese
- 1 cup mayonnaise or salad dressing
- 1/2 cup sour cream

To make:

Combine sour cream and Salad Dressing and thin slightly with milk till consistency of a thick salad dressing.

Combine all remaining ingredients and toss together in bowl.

Pour salad dressing over and toss lightly.

Allow to sit in refrigerator so that your flavors can begin to blend slightly before you serve the salad.

Hearty Summer Salad

Brunch or summertime meals can be difficult for those who are gluten intolerant or eat a gluten free diet. Cookouts often   mean that you're getting foods such as hamburgers which incorporate gluten laden ingredients and may also require buns. Gluten free can be a bit more difficult when trying to whip up a cool and easy summertime meal which doesn't require a lot of cooking.

This chickpea and black eyed pea salad is amazingly healthy and refreshing for those days when you just can't even look at the stove. High in protein and in fiber, you'll be well nourished while getting a break from the day to day cooking grind on those hot summer days.

You will need:

- 2 of the 15 oz. cans chickpeas
- 2 of the15 oz. cans black-eyed peas
- 2-15 oz. cans artichoke hearts
- 4 large tomatoes
- ½ large onion
- 3 large fresh garlic cloves
- ¼ cup olive oil
- ½ cup balsamic vinegar

- A few pinches parsley
- Fresh ground salt
- Pepper to taste
- 1/4 cup green olives
- 1/4 teaspoon dried basil

To make:

Drain the beans and add to a bowl.

Chop the artichoke hearts into 8 pieces each and add to the mixture.

Chop tomatoes or dice them into pieces.

Dice your onion and add to the mixture.

Crush the garlic and mince it very finely.

Drain olives and add to the mixture.

Chop the parsley finely.

Add the basil.

Mix your vinegar and olive oil To make a lovely topping.

Drizzle the dressing over the top.

Allow to cool in the refrigerator to blend your flavors for about an hour.

Appetizers and Snacks

It's difficult at times to find gluten free snacks and treats that you can serve at the afternoon Super Bowl Party or just for a quick snack. Most of the processed foods have come into contact with gluten in some way. If you're concerned about making sure that you're not going to be touched by a gluten product or you'd simply like to know how To make your own gluten free treats for a party, we've got a special section of snacks and appetizers for you to create.

Chicken wings are one of our favorite treats. If you're like us, the taste is great and a few of those delectable little bites are just right for an afternoon snack or a small finger food to be served up while you watch the big game. Two different varieties of chicken wings, each of them gluten free are offered here.

Our Chicken Wing recipes have it all. Great taste, lower fat, and just the right amount of heat.

Garlic and Parmesan Chicken Wings

You will need:

- One small can parmesan cheese (8 ounces)
- 1 teaspoon garlic powder
- 2 teaspoons sea salt, ground finely
- 1 stick margarine
- 1/2 teaspoon pepper
- 2 tablespoons corn meal
- 4 pounds chicken wings, cut up into pieces, with tips discarded

To make:

Preheat oven to 400 degrees

Place all ingredients except the margarine and chicken wings into a plastic zip lock bag

Shake to blend ingredients.

Lightly roll chicken wing into margarine and dip into the seasoning.

Place on foil lined cookie or baking sheet.

Sprinkle remaining seasonings over the top of your chicken wings and drizzle with margarine.

Bake at 400 until browned and completely done, approximately 30 minutes in preheated oven.

Test with meat thermometer to ensure proper temperature.

Hot and Spicy Chicken Wings

A little on the spicy side, you'll want to ensure that you have some milk or tomato juice on hand for those who may be affected by the heat in these.

You will need:

- 2 ounces of Louisiana hot sauce or hot pepper sauce
- 1/4 cup of ketchup
- 1/4 cup brown sugar
- 1 stick butter
- 1 teaspoon garlic powder
- sea salt grinder
- freshly ground pepper

To make:

Layer chicken wings on foil covered baking sheet. Brush lightly with butter and season to taste with salt and pepper.

Mix the remaining ingredients together and thoroughly brush over chicken wings.

Bake at 400 approximately 30-40 minutes until done

through.

Tips on "Snackable" Treats

Did you know that the FDA of the United States considers that fruits which have been frozen are comparable in nutrition to those which are fresh and they allow frozen fruit to be labeled as fresh fruit and considered to be healthy. Frozen fruit is already washed and is ready to eat.

Fruit is naturally gluten free and the cleaning the prepping has already been done for you. To enjoy a fast To make treat, take several of your favorites and add them to a smoothie. The phytonutrients as well as the fiber are incredibly good for you, in some cases even helping to detox the body and to give you some amazing nutrients and health benefits. Many fruits actually help to fight cancers of various types and can be used to protect your long term health.

Fruit is gluten free in most cases and it's just plain good for you. Snack on some fresh fruit or even frozen in order to stave off hunger and get a fast and easy gluten free snack.

Gluten Free Conserves and Relishes

Sometimes it's difficult to buy things like cranberry sauce and various types of relish which are not gluten free or aren't guaranteed not to have come into contact with gluten on machinery. Making your own eliminates that risk and gives you a fresher and more delicious product. One of the hardest things to find is a relish that doesn't have additives or glutens such as you will find in many of the different processed relishes and conserves. It's easy to create your own from fresh fruits and vegetables as well as to add other ingredients which are healthy and natural. Why take a chance on the jarred or canned items when you can make your own very easily and in a relatively short amount of time.

Raw Salsa

Salsa is one of our favorite things. Having had some contact with other ethnic groups over time, we've found that most Hispanics do not use the kind of salsa that we do, but rather make it fresh and raw at nearly every meal. We became very accustomed to this kind of salsa and really prefer it to the jarred variety. This recipe for raw salsa is heart healthy, free of gluten and absolutely delicious.

Home Made Spicy Salsa

You will need:

- 6 Roma or other meaty tomatoes
- 6 green onions
- 2 cloves of garlic
- 1 jalapeno
- 1 can chopped green chilies
- Handful of chopped cilantro
- 1 chopped bell pepper
- 1 teaspoon fresh lime juice
- 1/4 teaspoon ground sea salt
- Dash of pepper

To make:

Chop the tomatoes into small squares.

Finely chop remaining ingredients except for the jalapeno and add to the mixture.

Determine how hot you would like your salsa to be. Add one quarter, one half or one full jalapeno, depending upon your preference for heat.

Remove the seeds and chop the pepper finely, adding the portion that you would like.

Refrigerate your salsa for about 2 hours to allow the flavors to blend nicely.

Cranberry Conserve

Cranberry conserve is an old style way to use cranberries. It's a great changeover from the old jellied cranberry sauce that many people serve at the holiday. In our house, there is no such thing as a cranberry sauce that comes from a can. The risk that some of these items have come in contact with gluten is one that we would prefer not to take.

While this is wonderful at the holidays, it's also a super addition to nearly any meal and tastes great when used on burgers for a fresh new style. This is an old Amish recipe which has been rewritten To make it a bit easier To make and to store.

You will need:

- 4 cups of fresh cranberries
- 2 large oranges-sliced
- 1 cup chopped raisins (* you may prefer the golden variety
- of raisins)
- 2 cups of water
- 3 cups pure cane sugar
- 1/2 cup chopped nuts (optional, and we normally omit

- these. If you know of anyone with a nut allergy, avoid them).

To make:

Slice the oranges and discard the seeds

Grind the fresh cranberries and oranges, in a blender or chopper

Transfer it to a heavy sauce pan and add the water.

Cook the fruit rather quickly on a higher fire, being careful to prevent scorching.

Add sugar and raisins. Cook the mix over medium to low heat, stirring the conserve very often, until it begins to thicken.

This freezes very well and can be kept in the refrigerator for up to 14 days.

Gluten Free Desserts - Yes, They Can be Healthy

Healthy gluten free desserts are recipes are much sought after. In many cases, getting chocolate means that it is accompanied by other things that those who need to stay strictly gluten free cannot eat. We can't stress enough that you are going to need to really review cans and ingredients to ensure that your cocoa and other items have not been made on shared equipment and in places where wheat or gluten is present in tiny amounts.

In many cases, although we're uncertain why it is so, the brand names will be made on shared equipment while those which are not major brands will be cleaner and less likely to have contaminants. Check every label carefully to ensure that your products are gluten free and have not had the chance of being contaminated by other products which may contain gluten.

Hot Chocolate Pudding

Not only delicious, but also quite healthy with its touch of cocoa powder, containing phytonutrients that are actually proven to combat some types of cancer, your dessert will be luscious and nutritional, while at the same time being gluten free.

Hot Chocolate pudding is one of the most delicious desserts that you're going to find. It's easy To make and takes about 15 minutes from start to finish.

You will need:

- 2/3 cup pure cane sugar
- 2 tablespoons of corn starch
- pinch of salt
- 1 and 1/2 cups canned milk
- 1 and 1/2 cups water
- 4 egg yolks, slightly beaten
- 1/2 tsp. real vanilla
- 6 ounce bar of Hershey's Dark chocolate
- 1 tsp. Hershey's cocoa

To make:

Combine your sugar, the corn starch and the salt.

Adding about a fourth of a cup of milk, make a very smooth paste-like substance.

Add the remainder of the milk and your egg yolks, stirring til completely blended.

Put the pan over medium heat stirring constantly until it begins to thicken.

Pour into dessert cups and allow to set up about ten minutes.

Transfer into refrigerator or serve warm with a bit of cocoa sifted lightly over the top.

FAST and Easy Gluten Free Rice Pudding

Rice pudding, particularly warm rice pudding is a favorite of nearly everyone who tastes it. Topped with cinnamon it becomes a very healthy ending to your gluten free meal.

You will need:

- 4 egg yolks
- 2/3 cup granulated sugar
- 3 cups of milk
- 2 tablespoons of corn starch
- 1/2 tsp. pure vanilla extract
- 1/4 cup raisins (optional)
- 3/4 cups of instant rice
- dash of cinnamon

To make the rice pudding:

Make the instant rice in the microwave according to package directions. When making it during the last minute of cooking drop in the raisins into the rice to steam and soften them.

In a saucepan, combine the cornstarch, the sugar, and the egg yolks.

Stir until smooth, adding a slight amount of milk as necessary to thin the mixture down to a smooth paste.

Add the remaining milk and stir to combine all ingredients.

Cook over low heat for approximately 12 minutes until the mixture thickens. Do not boil.

Remove from heat and allow cooling approximately 5 minutes.

Drain any remaining water from the rice and raisins.

Combine the rice with the pudding mixture and spoon into dessert dishes.

Dust the top with cinnamon if desired.

Chocolate Fondue Dessert

Dark chocolate has made some big news recently for the fact that it is one of the newest--and the most taste tempting heart healthy foods. Dark chocolate keeps more of the flavonoids than the other varieties. New research is telling us that dark chocolate with its flavonoid content can help to keep your heart healthy and to prevent some types of cardiovascular diseases. Fortunately dark chocolate, which is rich in flavonoids is not rich in gluten--and remains one of the most delicious foods that you can eat which is gluten free.

Obviously that doesn't mean that you can ignore the high calorie content and dash to the store to get yourself a ton of dark chocolate to the exclusion of other kinds of food, but it does mean that when eaten in moderation as part of a healthy diet, dark chocolate can help you to stay healthier in the long term.

Dark Chocolate Fondue

You will need:

- 12 ounces Dark Chocolate finely chopped
- 3/4 cup heavy Whipping Cream

- Fresh strawberries
- Fresh pineapple
- Fresh blueberries
- Sliced bananas
- Fresh sliced apples

To make:

Heat the whipping cream until very warm and drop the chocolate into the whipping cream.

Allow all chocolate to melt thoroughly and stir til smooth, but do not allow boiling.

Keep warm over a pot of warm water in a double boiler and using toothpicks or bamboo skewers and dip the fresh fruit into the chocolate pot.

Gluten Free Chocolate Cake

Also called by some, gluten free soufflé, this is one of
the most decadent desserts that you will create which is
gluten free. One taste and you're absolutely in love.
Much more like a chocolate soufflé than it is a cake; the
taste is out of this world. The cocoa adds some
antioxidants to your dessert, keeping you healthier and
helping to stave off some long term disease processes.

You will need:

- 2 sticks of butter (you must use real butter for this
  recipe, not margarine which is slightly more
  watery)
- 1/4 cup Hershey's unsweetened cocoa, plus one
  teaspoon for dusting the pan
- 8 ounces of bitter, mildly sweetened chocolate,
  chopped into fine pieces
- 5 eggs
- 1 and 1/4 cups heavy whipping cream
- 1 cup pure cane sugar
- 1/2 cup sour cream
- 1/4 cup powdered sugar

To create the cake:

Preheat your oven to 350 degrees Fahrenheit

Butter a spring form pan measuring 9 inches.

Melt the butter and combine with the quarter cup of heavy cream until it is all melted.

Add the chocolate bars and allow melting. Stir to smooth the mixture and remove it from the heat.

Beat eggs, sugar and cocoa into the chocolate into the buttered pan, add the batter you've just created and bake until the entire mixture is set and puffed up. It will take about 40 minutes to cook completely.

Allow to cool approximately 40 minutes to an hour before you try to unmold the cake.

Beat the sour cream and the confectioners' sugar with the remaining heavy cream and serve as a sauce.

Decadent does not even begin to describe this dessert, which is lovely enough to serve to guests at a holiday dinner.

Baked Apples

With walnuts which are heart healthy, as well as the cinnamon, these can be a healthy part of your diet. Walnuts which contain the omega fatty acids are a good part of a healthy diet. Desserts don't have to be unhealthy. While the butter adds a small amount of saturated fat to your diet, it is so slight as to be negligible.

You will need:

- 4 apples, preferably Cortland or Spies
- 1/4 cup brown sugar
- 5 teaspoons water
- 1/4 teaspoon cinnamon
- 2 tbsp. real butter, cut into slices
- Walnuts or pecans for garnish, as desired

To make baked apples:

Preheat the oven to 375 degrees.

Core the apples, removing the seeds and slice the bottom off so that they lay flat in the baking dish.

Place each apple in the pan.

Drop a small pat of butter inside each apple.

Mix the brown sugar and the water To make a slightly thick syrup.

Drip the syrup over the apples and bake them for approximately 20-30 minutes.

Take the sauce from the dish and spoon over the warm apple.

Serve with ice cream or whipped cream if desired.

Coffee Chocolate Mousse

Chocolate mousse is another of those decadent dessert treats that will leave you feeling very satisfied. You're not going to know that you're missing gluten at all with desserts like these, which make wonderful desserts for dinner parties or for the perfect holiday meal.

You will need:

- One Hershey's Special (tm) dark bar 8 ounce size
- 3 egg yolks, slightly beaten
- 2 teaspoons instant coffee
- 6 tablespoons sugar
- 2 cups whipping cream

To create the mousse:

Melt your chocolate into a bowl over water or in a double boiler. Stir once in a while until smooth.

In a small pan, whip your egg yolks, coffee powder and 3/4 cup of the whipping cream, as well as 4 tbsp. of granulated sugar.

Heat thoroughly, stirring all the while for about three minutes, but do not allow the mixture to completely boil.

Add the mixture to the chocolate mixture, stirring until smooth and glossy.

Cool completely, refrigerating if necessary for about half an hour.

Using your mixer beat the cream and the remaining sugar until it is forming stiff peaks.

Fold in one third of the chocolate mix, then the second, and finally the third portion of it.

Pour into glass serving bowls and refrigerate until hard.

If desired, garnish with shaved chocolate or sifted cocoa powder.

Gluten Free Tips for Fun Kid Foods

It's difficult to have a child who requires a gluten free diet. In many cases, like their friends, they want to eat "normal" foods which can cause them some long term health problems. If you're one of the millions of moms who have a child requiring a gluten free diet, you can't change what they need, but you can change it To make their diet a bit more fun and interesting.

These ideas are based on some fun facts and some fun ideas for moms which can make meal time just a bit less of a struggle.

Gluten Free Breakfast Idea

Remember the old Dr. Seuss Books. One that was always a favorite was "Green Eggs and Ham." Make a child's sleepover a lot more fun and cover the fact that your child isn't eating the typical cereal by making a healthy and a fun breakfast of Green Eggs and Ham.

Just a few drops of food coloring will create a very

festive meal of green eggs and ham, keeping your child--and his or her prospective company--away from the fact that there are not the typical sugary cereals at the breakfast table. Additionally you're adding some real nutritional value and keeping them clear of high sugar breakfast foods.

To turn scrambled eggs green, you'll want to use blue food coloring, while the green works well on the ham (turkey ham is better). Just a drop will do the job.

Gluten Free Chocolate Chip Cookies

Kids love chocolate chip cookies, but finding one that is gluten free and allows your child to enjoy the treats that other kids take for granted isn't always an easy task. Even some chocolate chips are processed on equipment that is not always free of the allergen that troubles them.

One answer to this is using buckwheat flour to create recipes. Despite its name, buckwheat is not true wheat. It is gluten free, according to the Celiac disease website and offers a lot of protein and iron on top of being gluten free.

Creating chocolate chip cookies from buckwheat, which is a good substitute for traditional flour makes them a tiny bit heavier but allows your kids to have the treat that they want, and you want to give them.

You will need:

- 1 and 1/4 cup buckwheat flour
- 1/2 tsp. soda
- 1/2 tsp. salt
- 1 stick of butter

- 1/4 cup dark brown sugar
- 1/2 tsp. vanilla extract
- 1 egg
- 1 cup chocolate chips (remember to check the package to ensure they are gluten free)

To make:

Combine the dry ingredients except the sugar

Whip together softened butter, egg and sugar

Mix the sugar mixture with the remaining dry ingredients and mix thoroughly.

Stir in chocolate chips

Drop by rounded teaspoons onto a lined cookie sheet.

Bake at 375 degrees for 9-12 minutes.

Crock Pot Cookery and Gluten Free?

One of the questions that is most frequently asked is can I make gluten free recipes in the crock pot. The answer to that is a resounding yes. Most soups and stews are naturally gluten free, using only meats and vegetables. Your favorite recipes of any kind can be made in the crock pot to give you some easy ways to create a meal ahead of time.

Adapting recipes for your slow cooker.

Whether you are cooking traditional foods or gluten free foods, there are times when you want to prepare your food ahead of time and have it ready to go when you arrive at home. In most cases, vegetable and meat stews are going to be easier to prepare and can be made ahead of time to be ready for a hot meal if you're using a crock pot. Soups and stews can have all of the preparation work accomplished the night before and be placed in the crock pot to cook away while you do other things.

Most recipes can be adapted for the crock pot, offering a great way to leave your hands free in meal preparation. The advantages of the crock pot are that they offer you better meals, which are going to be healthier in nature and lower in fats than most of the fast food choices you might make.

Here are a few tips for changing your recipes to crock pot ready recipes.

Bear in mind that if you're going to be using frozen veggies, they only need about half hour, so add them to your recipes for the last 40 minutes of cooking.

Soak dried items such as beans or lentils for an hour or so prior to adding them to the crock pot.

If the recipes require pasta, even gluten free pasta, that too should only be added in the last hour of cooking time.

Bear in mind that you want to lower the liquid amounts in crock pot cooking. You will want to lower them by about one quarter of the overall liquid recipe since the lid doesn't allow for a vast amount of evaporation.

When using the crock pot, layering the veggies on the

bottom and adding the meat to the top is the best plan of action.

If your recipe takes about 30 minutes cook time, it will take about 3 hours on high, 4 hours on medium, and 6 hours on low in the crock pot.

Restaurant Foods on a Gluten Free Diet

Eating out always has the potential to be difficult, but it can be particularly so when you are on any type of a restricted diet. Typically any meal that offers gravy is going to use a roux to thicken it, so make sure that you ask before you order that Sunday roast at a restaurant.

Many places today cater to gluten free people and do have a special menu that they can offer which allows for gravy and sauces which are made from corn flour rather than roux as a thickening agent.

Prior to heading out to a new restaurant a phone call may be in order to find out what kind of foods are available on the menu rather than hoping you find something you may be able to eat and finding out that you're wrong.

Nearly every restaurant serves fresh fruit of some type, but you'll want to be sure there is something else there that you can make a meal of rather than leaving it to chance.

If you find yourself in a restaurant on the spur of the moment, there are some foods that usually do not require the addition of anything which may be gluten laden.

Some choices that you can make which are typically gluten free in the restaurants (although do ask to be sure) include:

- Roast turkey
- Broiled Chicken
- Pork Chops
- Broiled Steaks
- Fresh steamed veggies

Desserts are going to be the most difficult to get when you are on a gluten free diet, but bear in mind that your selections can include fruit salads, as well as crème brulee, along with nearly any type of pudding which is typically made with corn flour as opposed to a flour thickening agent.

Make sure that you ask your server and if you do not get a satisfactory answer, do ask to speak with the chef in order to find out what kind of gluten free menu items the restaurant offers.

Tips on Living Gluten Free:

1. Many foods are naturally gluten free. You do not have to shop the fringe to find all gluten free foods. Things like rice noodles, buckwheat, fruits and veggies are gluten free naturally. Use those products and save some money on the cost of buying gluten free.

2. Use common sense. Many companies make a big production and a big payday by touting their foods as gluten free. There is even a gluten free rice. The rice grain is naturally gluten free so make sure you are aware of what foods are gluten free before paying more for a product that may be naturally gluten free.

3. Many stores carry a list of foods that are gluten free. Bigger shopping sites such as Trader Joe's, Wegmans and many other supermarkets will be glad to give you a list of gluten free goods and enable you To make great choices without searching the entire store.

4. Make sure you look for "gluten free" on the label. Gluten free and wheat free are two entirely different things and not all products which are free of wheat are also free of gluten.

5. Buy a few good books. Richard Coppedge, Jr, who is a professor of baking and pastry arts at The Culinary Institute of America is also the author of a book on gluten free baking that may become your new Bible. " Gluten-Free Baking With The Culinary Institute of America: 150 Flavorful Recipes From the World's Premier Culinary College.

6. Some types of oil may have been made on equipment which was shared with gluten containing products. Check the labels of everything, even those foods which you believe should be gluten free. It doesn't hurt to be a little extra careful.

7. Many companies today make foods which are already done and are gluten free. Check them for use in those moments when you need something fast and easy. Gluten free premade meals are available in most regular supermarkets today.

8. Online websites are one of the best places to find gluten free tips and new gluten free recipes. In fact, at last count there were about 5000 gluten free recipe sites which can be used to help you to supplement your meals and to get great substitutions for foods or products that contain gluten.

9. If you live in a small area, supermarkets and even companies such as Amazon are offering online gluten free products that you can order. Typically the shipping prices are quite low and you'll have the products within just a few days. If you live in an area where the supermarket is not large and gluten free products aren't part of what they carry, shopping online can be a life-saver.

10. Rice flour is amazing for fried foods. While it is gritty and often causes problems in bread, the rice flour for use when frying items or making tempura is a wonderful addition because that bit of extra texture is very welcome. Don't rule out rice flour all together when you're cooking because of the grit.

References and Credits

We've made several statements during the course of the book which promote the use of broccoli, cauliflower, and other cruciferous vegetables being used in gluten free cooking to aid in detoxifying the body and to assist in adding fiber to the diet. These statements are made using references from the Pub Med materials and the Nutritional Journal references which can be found below.

Ambrosone CB, Tang L. Cruciferous vegetable intake and cancer prevention: role of nutrigenetics. Cancer Prev Res (Phila Pa). 2009 Apr;2(4):298-300.

Angeloni C, Leoncini E, Malaguti M, et al. Modulation of phase II enzymes by sulforaphane: implications for its cardioprotective potential. J Agric Food Chem. 2009 Jun 24;57(12):5615-22.

Banerjee S, Wang Z, Kong D, et al. 3,3'-Diindolylmethane enhances chemosensitivity of multiple chemotherapeutic agents in pancreatic cancer. 3,3'-Diindolylmethane enhances chemosensitivity of multiple chemotherapeutic agents in pancreatic cancer.

Bhattacharya A, Tang L, Li Y, et al. Inhibition of bladder cancer development by allyl isothiocyanate. Carcinogenesis. 2010 Feb;31(2):281-6.

Bryant CS, Kumar S, Chamala S, et al. Sulforaphane induces cell cycle arrest by protecting RB-E2F-1 complex in epithelial ovarian cancer cells. Molecular Cancer 2010, 9:47.

Christopher B, Sanjeez K, Sreedhar C, et al. Sulforaphane induces cell cycle arrest by protecting RB-E2F-1 complex in epithelial ovarian cancer cells. Molecular Cancer Year: 2010 Vol: 9 Issue: 1 Pages/record No.: 47.

Clarke JD, Dashwood RH, Ho E. Multi-targeted prevention of cancer by sulforaphane. Cancer Lett. 2008 Oct 8;269(2):291-304.

Cornelis MC, El-Sohemy A, Campos H. GSTT1 genotype modifies the association between cruciferous vegetable intake and the risk of myocardial infarction. Am J Clin Nutr. 2007 Sep;86(3):752-8.

Hu J, Straub J, Xiao D, et al. Phenethyl isothiocyanate, a cancer chemopreventive constituent of cruciferous vegetables, inhibits cap-dependent translation by regulating the level and phosphorylation of 4E-BP1. Cancer Res. 2007 Apr 15;67(8):3569-73.

Jiang H, Shang X, Wu H, et al. Combination treatment with resveratrol and sulforaphane induces apoptosis in human U251 glioma cells. Neurochem Res. 2010 Jan;35(1):152-61.

Special Thanks to WHFoods for their valuable information on broccoli, cauliflower and other cruciferous vegetables as well as the reference materials to point us in the right direction.

The American Journal of Clinical Nutrition was an invaluable resource in the creation of this book. Find them online at http://ajcn.nutrition.org/

Section 2: Gluten Free Vegan

It seems as if every time you turn around there is another diet plan being touted as the miracle answer to all that ails you, especially excessive weight. Gluten free and vegan diets do not necessarily fall into this category! Each has become progressively more popular, however the reasons behind this type of lifestyle change goes far beyond losing weight.

There are many different reasons people consider drastic changes to their diet and lifestyle. Many times health is a major motivator, especially when it comes to eliminating gluten from your daily diet. Here are a few common reasons individuals choose to live a gluten free vegan lifestyle:

- You are a vegan and discovered you have gluten intolerance or celiac disease
- You are concerned with the ethical treatment of animals slaughtered for meat production
- You want a healthier diet filled with rich, live foods (plants do not have to die to provide a meal.)
- Meat and processed foods are expensive

- You have suffered various ailments over the years that are only alleviated with a gluten free diet

If you have been considering this shift in eating habits, you should understand what it means to be vegan and how gluten can cause various issues for someone who is sensitive to wheat proteins.

Gluten

Gluten is a protein found in foods processed from wheat and related grains. Many people are shocked to learn just how many items at the grocery store contain gluten or are gluten contaminated. For many people this is not a big deal, but for those who suffer from gluten sensitivity or celiac disease, it is a very big deal indeed.

Celiac Disease

In many circles the use of the phrases gluten intolerance and celiac disease are used interchangeably, however recent research suggests intolerance may have a much broader scope than celiac disease. To date, however, many medical journals may use the terms interchangeably.

What is gluten intolerance or celiac disease? If you are sensitive to gluten the sensitive villi in your digestive tract can become damaged when you consume gluten laden products via an allergic type reaction in which the immune system attacks the lining of your digestive tract. The exact cause of the disease is unknown and can develop at any age.

Symptoms:

- Abdominal pain- bloating, gas or heartburn
- Nausea and vomiting
- Changes in appetite (up or down)
- Foul stool that floats, appears fatty or shows evidence of blood
- Depression
- Hair loss
- Skin rashes
- Joint pain and aches
- Brain fog
- Chronic constipation
- Fatigue
- Changes to menstrual cycle
- Stunted growth
- Tingling or numbness in hands and feet

It is important to note that these are but a few symptoms, not a comprehensive list. Furthermore you may suffer few, many or be completely asymptomatic.

If all of this is sounding familiar, you may want to begin the diagnostic process with a self test, which is really just asking yourself some basic questions related to major symptoms. If you are dealing with four or more symptoms, it is time to talk to your physician as you may have a gluten sensitivity issue. Your doctor will want to run a series of tests to confirm your diagnosis, before you change your eating habits.

Vegan Lifestyle and Diet

Vegan and vegetarian are quite similar, but with a few pronounced differences. Some would say that a vegan diet is merely a stricter form of vegetarianism, and to some extent that is true. However, practitioners feel a vegan lifestyle is as much a philosophy as it is a diet plan.

History

Vegetarianism has been around since at least the 19th century, and the first vegan cookbook was published in 1910. Nevertheless, the word vegan was not coined until 1944 when a couple members of the Leicester Vegetarian Society expressed concern over the fact that vegetarians were still consuming dairy products. The first vegan society in the United States was founded in 1948.

Philosophy

Veganism has a "mission" (for lack of a better phrase) statement that sum up this particular groups beliefs and motivations.

"The doctrine that man should live without exploiting animals." This means that in addition to meat being stricken from the menu, for example:

- Meat- (goes without saying)
- Eggs- it is a baby chicken after all
- Honey- bees are taken advantage of for human consumption.

Concern for the ethical treatment of farm animals is but one reason people turn to a vegan lifestyle. Recent studies suggest a cause and effect relationship between the consumption of red meat and increased incidences of colon cancer. Add to that the concerns about growth hormones in chicken and the use of a multitude of drugs in cattle, pork and chickens, it is not really difficult to see why more and more people are second guessing their diets and lifestyles.

Of course, opting for a vegan diet, particularly one that is gluten free is not exactly easy! However, with the right recipes and a little encouragement you will soon find yourself on the way to a healthier and more environmentally friendly life.

Gluten Free Vegan Alternative Ingredients

One of the biggest challenges with a gluten free vegan diet is finding recipes that are tasty and satisfying. The list of prohibited foods is long, but you can still create delicious meals and even some family favorites by substituting ingredients and learning to use fragrant spices and colorful vegetables in your dishes. Let's start by discussing some vegan and gluten free substitutes for popular ingredients.

Eggs

Eggs are a great source of protein and a common binding agent in a myriad of recipes. Thankfully, you can use several replacement ingredients, depending on the type of dish you are creating. A few examples include:

Sweet Dishes- Cakes, cookies and other desserts

- Applesauce- ¼ cup for each egg
- Vinegar and Baking powder- when you have a

recipe calling for three or more eggs, you can use this substitute: 1 tablespoon each vinegar, water and baking powder.

- Potato Starch- 2 heaping tablespoons
- Pureed banana- ¼ cup per egg (for lighter cakes the conversion is 3 tablespoons per egg)
- Water- ¼ cup per egg
- Soy Yogurt- ¼ per egg
- Arrowroot- 2 heaping teaspoons per egg
- Binding Agents- non-desert recipes
- 2-3 Tablespoons- mashed potato flakes, arrowroot powder or tomato paste
- Vegetable Oil- ¼ cup per egg
- Flax Seed- 1 tablespoon ground seed to 3 tablespoons of water (great source of omega 3's)

Flour

If you like to bake cakes, cookies and breads you will need gluten free flour substitutes. You might be inclined to think you can just grab a gluten free alternative off the shelf and substitute it cup for cup in your favorite recipe, however it is not quite that simple. Gluten free alternatives have different textures, flavors and fat contents. For example coconut flour absorbs water like crazy and almond flour has a distinct flavor.

A good alternative is to create your own all-purpose flour mixture.

Alternative Flour Mixture:

1 ½ cup millet flour
1 ½ cup sorghum flour
1 ¾ cup potato starch

As you begin creating your own dishes you will probably want to tinker with the above mixture, feel free to mix and match ingredients and amounts until you find the perfect all-purpose flour alternative for your favorite dishes.

Gluten Free Flours

Bean Flours:

- Kinako- roasted soy flour
- Garbanzo bean
- Fava bean
- White Flours
- Sweet rice
- White rice
- Tapioca

- Nut Flours
- Coconut
- Almond
- Chestnut
- Whole Grain
- Brown rice
- Quinoa
- Teff

In the beginning your recipes will be more like mini-adventures, but that is half the fun! Why make gluten free vegan living a boring endeavor? If you happen to opt for dark buckwheat as a gluten free flour alternative, you should know your dish will have a decided purple hue.

Butter

Butter has several roles in baking, it can act as a binding agent, leavening agent, adds flavor and sometimes texture. However, since it is a dairy product it must be stricken from the vegan shopping list. Thankfully it is fairly easy to replace. Here are a few options:

Butter to Olive Oil:

1 teaspoon- ¾ teaspoon

1 tablespoon- 2 ¼ teaspoon

¼ cup- 3 tablespoons

For cookies or recipes where creamed butter is required coconut oil is a better option. You can use identical quantities and then simply beat the coconut butter to a semi-solid state. Other butter substitutes include but are not limited to:

Untoasted sesame seed oil

Vegan shortening

Canola oil

Milk Substitutes

Probably one of the easiest substitutions to make today as there are already a number of non-dairy alternatives available at your local grocery store. A few you might want to consider include:

Almond Milk

Soy Milk

Coconut milk

Non-dairy powdered milk

Meat Substitutes

Not all vegans are interested in substituting for meat, however if you would still like the occasional burger or do not fancy spaghetti with sauce alone, you may want some alternatives. One thing you have to watch with popular commercial vegan meat substitutes is the wheat content. For the gluten free vegan diet, you will have to stick with soy and tofu based alternatives, but make sure you read the ingredients list. Tofu is generally the go to meat replacement as it is basically tasteless and will take on the flavor of whatever seasonings you use in your dish.

Now that you have some idea of what you should add to your shopping list, it is time to get on with some tasty recipes! Here are a few tried and tested gluten free vegan recipes you can add to your recipe caddy.

Vegan Pasta

2 cups chickpea flour
12 tablespoons water
4 tablespoons ground flaxseed

Mix together flaxseed and warm water, gently whisk ingredients together and set aside. On your cutting /

rolling board, pour your chickpea flour, making a mound of sorts. Create a well in the center. Once the flaxseed mixture has jelled, (five minutes or so) pour in the middle of your flour well.

Mix chickpea flour and flaxseed together gently, forming a dough ball. Wrap in plastic wrap and allow to sit at room temperature for approximately half an hour.

The key to making tasty pasta with chickpea flour is getting the dough rolled thin enough, which can be a challenge. If you plan to do this the old fashioned way, (roller and countertop) make sure to use small portions of the dough at a time. Roll very thin, cut into squares and create bowtie pasta. (Easiest pasta form to make without a pasta machine)

Gluten Free Vegan Pie Crust

1 ½ cup rice flour or other gluten free alternative (some flours will be sweeter than others)
½-cup shortening- (may substitute vegan margarine)
4 tablespoons water

Create dough balls by cutting shortening or alternative into the flour until you have a crumbly mixture. Gently form into balls and then either roll flat with your rolling pin or form it to your pie pan by hand. Bake in oven for 10-15 minutes at 400 degrees.

Gluten Free Vegan Recipes

Snacks

No matter how healthy your diet may be, snacks are probably a part of your daily routine. If not, once you get a load of these tasty, yet gluten free vegan alternatives, you will change your mind.

Onion Rings

If onion rings are your sole purpose for hitting the fast food drive through, you are in luck with this first snack. Not only is it easy to prepare and cost effective, it tastes great and you can enjoy it any time day or night from the comfort of your own home.

1 med onion- sweet Vidalia's are a good option
¼ cup soy milk (almond works as well)
½ cup coconut flour
Season to Taste- cayenne pepper, salt, garlic seasoning, onion powder etc...

Slice your onion carefully, laying aside intact rings. Place milk and flour in separate bowls, adding your preferred seasonings to the flour. Dip each ring first in milk and then in the flour, being careful to fully coat each ring. Lay rings separately on a non-stick baking pan. Bake for 20 minutes at 450°.

Sweet Potato Fries

McDonald's may have some of the best French fries on the market today, but they cannot hold a candle to sweet potato fries! Healthy and great tasting, why opt for a greasy high calorie alternative?

1-3 medium sweet potatoes
1-2 teaspoons coconut oil
1 tablespoon equal parts cinnamon/ sugar (check labels for gluten free processed spices)

Peel and slice sweet potatoes, making strips of raw potatoes (fries). Place fries in a single layer on a non-stick baking sheet. Drizzle fries with coconut oil and sprinkle lavishly with sugar/ cinnamon mixture. Bake fries for approximately 30 minutes at 425°. For added snacking pleasure dust warm fries with powdered sugar.

Peanut Butter Apple (quick snack)

Sometimes you want a tasty snack but do not have the time to slice, cook and wait! For those occasions sliced apples and a peanut butter dip can really hit the spot.

½ cup peanut butter
Dash of coconut milk
Pinch of cinnamon

First, choose your apples, Fuji and gala are probably the most common peel and eat apples, but if you like, something with a bit more bite a granny smith will work.

In a medium mixing bowl combine ingredients and beat on medium speed until your peanut butter dip is nice and creamy. Peel, core and slice your apples. Voila, you have a tasty snack you can whip up in a hurry.

TIP: If you are in a big hurry a couple tablespoons of peanut butter in a dish makes a great dip for apples. Better than caramel covered apples any day of the week!

Main Dishes

The real challenge on a gluten free vegan diet is the main course. Snacks and sides are fairly simple as you can always choose from a variety of in season fruits and vegetables. Here are a few main dishes you can experiment with.

Vegetables and Rice

This is a delicious filling main dish and keeping it gluten free and vegan friendly couldn't be simpler.

2 cups uncooked rice

2 medium onions

2 carrots

2 tomatoes or 14 oz. can of stewed tomatoes

3 whole cloves of garlic

3 celery stalks (no leaves)

1 bay leaf (optional)

Salt and pepper to taste

Sit rice and tomatoes aside, separately. Begin preparations by chopping onions, carrots and celery into medium to large chunks. Place all vegetables in stock pot and add enough water to completely cover. Next add garlic, cloves and a dash of salt and pepper. Bring water and vegetables to a boil over high heat, then reduce heat and simmer for 45 minutes to an hour. About half way through add stewed tomatoes to the mix.

When vegetables are soft but not mushy, remove from heat and strain 3-4 cups of broth. Place rice in a medium sized pan, cover with vegetable broth and cook according to type of rice. Serve vegetables on bed of fragrant rice and enjoy!

NOTE: You can add other vegetables as the fancy strikes, potatoes, peas and even corn can create a colorful and tasty dish. You can also alter garlic and onion amounts to suit your personal preferences.

Chickpea Salad

Gluten free and vegan friendly this little salad is chock full of protein and fiber, which means it, is a salad that will stick with you until dinnertime. This makes a perfect light, yet healthy lunch alternative.

2 cups Chickpeas- cooked
1 oz. olive oil
1 large cucumber- sliced
1/3 cup of fresh dill- finely chopped
1 lemon- juice and zest

Place dry chickpeas in a large bowl, completely cover with water and allow to soak overnight. Drain chickpeas, place in a large pot or stock pan and add four cups of water. (Water is always double the amount of chickpeas). Bring to a boil over high heat, reduce temperature and cook for approximately one hour or until chickpeas are done to your personal preference. Place in bowl, top with sliced cucumber and set aside.

Combine dill, lemon juice and zest in a mixing bowl and whisk together, creating a tasty dressing for your chickpea and cucumber salad.

Pasta Marinara

Who doesn't love a big bowl of pasta on occasion?
Thankfully, today's gluten free pasta's taste much better
than they used to! Remember the days when you could
not be sure if you were eating the noodles or the box?
No more my friend!

8 oz. dry gluten free vegan pasta
1 cup chopped green bell pepper
1 cup chopped onion
3 cloves garlic- minced
½ cup chopped celery
½ cup chopped carrots
4 tablespoons olive oil
6 oz. tomato paste
14-16 oz. can tomatoes
1-teaspoon dry oregano
1-teaspoon dry basil
½-teaspoon dry thyme
1-teaspoon sugar
½-cup water

Heat oil in a large skillet and cook together until tender
carrots, garlic, onion, celery and peppers. Add tomatoes,
spices, tomato paste, ½-cup water and sugar. Bring
entire mixture to a boil the reduce heat, cover and

simmer ½ hour. Stir occasionally, checking for desired consistency.

Follow packaged directions for preparing your particular brand of gluten free pasta. Most pasta is best served al dente. Cook pasta, drain, add marinara sauce and serve. Serves 4-6 people.

Possible Gluten Free Pasta Option:

Gluten free pasta is a bit easier to find than vegan-gluten free pasta! When all else fails you can make your own!

Simple Mexican Stew

If you thought you would have to give up your favorite type of food to stay on a gluten free vegan path, think again. Mexican stew is easy to make and delicious too!

16 oz. cupful brown beans
4 onions
4 potatoes
6 tomatoes
4 Tablespoon sugar
2 cups grape-juice
2-lemon rind
Water
2-teaspoon cumin
1-teaspoon paprika
1-teaspoon chili powder

Soak beans in approximately 10 cups of water for around 12 hours, overnight usually works. Chop vegetables into bite sized chunks. Add all ingredients to stockpot with beans and simmer for about an hour.

Simple Spanish Rice

Just in case you want a little something extra to go with you Mexican stew. Spanish rice is very simple to make, though there are dozens of alternatives to this particular recipe.

½-pound rice
1 can rotel
8 oz. tomato sauce
1-teaspoon ground cumin
½-teaspoon chili powder
½-teaspoon paprika

Cook rice according to package instructions, combine remaining ingredients adjusting spices to your personal preferences. Always strive to keep cumin levels higher than chili powder, unless you want a nice pan of "chili" rice. After adding tomato sauce, rotel and spices warm slightly over low heat, remember to stir this mixture well especially while warming.

NOTE: Do not be afraid to tinker with the spices, if you will remember to keep the cumin levels slightly higher than the chili powder and paprika you will always get a taco like flavor. You can also add some nice fresh corn for added flavor, color and deliciousness!

Vegetable Pot Pie

Do you recall those lovely little pot pies grandma used to pop in the oven when you were little? Enjoy this comfort food all over again with a tasty gluten free vegan alternative. Enjoy the memories of childhood while maintaining your diet.

1 T olive oil
3 carrots peeled
2 stalks celery
1 red bell pepper
1 medium onion, diced
1-cup fresh peas
1 clove minced garlic
2 new potatoes- chopped or diced small
1/2 cup dry white wine
1/2 cup gluten-free flour
2 cups mushroom stock
1-cup non-dairy milk (soy, coconut, almond, etc...)
1 T sage- roughly chopped

Take half a tablespoon of olive oil, place in medium saucepan over high heat. Stir in carrots, celery, bell pepper, garlic, potatoes and onion. Cook over medium high heat for approximately five minutes. Pour in white wine and reduce heat, cook for another 15 minutes. In a separate saucepan, use the other half of the olive oil to sauté your mushrooms.

Combine sautéed mushrooms and other vegetables together, add mushroom stock (vegetable stock works well also), peas and sage. Sprinkle all of the ingredients with gluten free flour. Stir to ensure flour breaks up nicely and add non-dairy milk. Cook over low heat for about 5 minutes, give or take. At this point, you are ready to transfer vegetable mixture to piecrust, shell.

Use the recipe above for gluten free vegan piecrust, make two balls of dough. Roll out and prepare two crusts, one to line the pie pan and the other for the top crust. Bake in a 425 degree oven for 10-15 minutes, reduce oven temperature to 325 and bake approximately one hour, or until crust is a golden brown.

Side Dishes

Potato Rice Balls

Do you want a side dish that will go with nearly any main course? Potato rice balls will do the trick nicely.

One large onion- finely chopped
Four large potatoes
One cup cooked rice
Olive oil

Cook potatoes and onions together until potatoes are mash able. Mash potatoes, mix in pre-cooked rice, season to taste and form into medium sized balls. Cook in large skillet with olive oil until heated through. For added flavor, green bell peppers and garlic make wonderful additions.

Vegan Baked Potato

Have you been wondering if you would ever have another delicious baked potato? If you crave a loaded baked potato covered in butter, cheese and sour cream, you are out of luck. However, if you want a fantastic tasting alternative that is good for you too, try this wonderful recipe.

2-3 medium to large russet potatoes
1 c broccoli florets
1 c cauliflower pieces
1 c carrots- matchstick
2 cloves chopped garlic
1/4 c apple juice, unsweetened
1 T lemon juice or balsamic vinegar
1/2- 1 tsp. lemon pepper
1 tsp. Italian Herb seasoning
Cooking Spray- olive oil preferably

Wash and wrap baking potatoes, place in 400-degree oven. Bake for approximately 20 minutes or until done.

While potatoes cook, combine cauliflower, carrots, broccoli, and garlic together. Spray generously with olive oil cooking spray. Add seasonings and toss with lemon juice and unsweetened apple juice. Place vegetables in a glass-baking dish, and cook on bottom rack of oven for about 40 minutes. Vegetables and potatoes should be fork tender when done.

Remove all from oven, split baked potato and garnish with vegetable mixture. For added pleasure top with a small amount of vegan grated parmesan cheese.

Chestnut Rissoles

Rissoles are a dish not unlike a meat loaf because basically anything goes! These were popular during and immediately after WWII as a way to make food, particularly meat go further. Leftover meats would be mixed with mashed potatoes, carrots, onions or anything that was available, then rolled in flour and fried for a tasty little cake. This is but one gluten free vegan rissole alternative.

1-pound Chestnuts
1 T chopped Parsley
1 T corn flour
1 T water

Cook chestnuts over medium high heat for about 30 minutes. Remove from stove, shell and mash nuts to form a paste. In a separate bowl combine cornmeal and water, mix well. Use the cornmeal mixture to moisten chestnut paste. Form rissole paste into small, rather flat pieces and roll in either vegan flour mixture or extra cornmeal. Fry in your choice of oils and serve.

Polenta and Corn

There are so many ways to prepare and use polenta; it has even been used as a noodle substitute for vegan lasagna! For today's busy families however, simpler is often best particularly when it comes to gluten free vegan diets.

2 c water
2 c unsweetened soymilk
1 tsp. salt
1 c cornmeal
1 T vegan buttery spread (earth balance is a good choice)
1/3 c unflavored, gluten-free soy creamer
2 tablespoons yeast (not brewer's yeast!)
1 1/2 c fresh corn

In a medium saucepan combine water, salt, and soymilk over medium heat, bring to a boil. Carefully whisk in cornmeal mixture and reduce heat. Stir constantly to remove lumps and prevent scorching, (about two minutes). Add vegan butter spread stirring until mixture is nice and creamy. Cook about 20 minutes, adding water if mix becomes to dry or thick.

When polenta has reached desired consistency stir in corn, yeast and soy creamer. You may need to cook mixture over low heat for a few more minutes after adding the last few ingredients.

Desserts

Zucchini Banana Spice Cake

Spice cake like mom used to make? On a gluten free vegan diet? Yes, yes you can! All it takes is a few minor alterations and you have a great desert you can enjoy morning, noon or night.

1 Pound Zucchini- peeled and grated (approximately 3 cups)
16 oz. flaked coconut
16 oz. walnuts- ground
12 tablespoons pureed banana
1 ½-cup tapioca starch flour
1 ½ cup white rice flour (mixing the two prevents a grainy texture)
1-teaspoon baking powder
1-teaspoon baking soda
2 teaspoons vanilla
2 ½ cups sugar
1 teaspoon of salt
Preheat oven 350°

Mix together coconut, walnuts and zucchini then set aside. Beat together pureed bananas, vanilla and oil in large mixing bowl. Beat in sugar and gradually add remaining dry ingredients, beating the mixture well. Add zucchini mixture, gently mix and pour into prepared cake pan/pans. (2-10 inch pans work well) Bake for 35-45 minutes. Allow to cool and frost to taste.

Creamy Apple Tapioca

An apple a day keeps the doctor away, and is there any better way to preserve your health? It may not be an apple fritter or cobbler, but it is quite tasty anyway.

1/2 cup tapioca
2-5 apples - approximately a pound
2 cups water
Sugar to taste
Lemon peel- grated yellow side
1 tsp. cinnamon (optional)

Preparations for this sweet dish begin the night before! Soak tapioca in 2 cups of water overnight. Peel, core and slice apples in quarters. In a medium sauce pan cook apples over medium low heat until they are nice and tender. Next, place them in a pie pan, sprinkle with sugar, grated part of lemon peel, and cinnamon (if you like). Finally mix in tapioca and water and bake for about an hour at 350 degrees. Remove from oven, serve chilled.

Strawberries in Cherry Syrup

If you are counting calories, you might want to skip this particular recipe! Nevertheless, if you do by chance have a skip day coming, try your hand at this delectable treat.

1-pound Strawberries
1-pound Cherries
2 C water
2 C granulated sugar

If you want to go really old school with this recipe, dust off your mortar and pestle! Start by grinding the cherries, pit and all, into a pasty substance. Place crushed cherries, water and sugar into a medium saucepan. Boil uncovered for one hour.

Strain cherry syrup into a smaller saucepan and reduce over medium heat until syrup begins to thicken. Remove from heat add strawberries to syrup and stir or shake around to thoroughly cover. Place strawberries on serving platter, return syrup to stove and cook for a few more minutes to thicken further. Drizzle remaining sauce over strawberries, allow to cool and enjoy!

Banana Nut Bread

An all-time favorite comfort food! If you thought you were going to have to give it up on your gluten free vegan diet, you will be very happy to find this recipe.

2 cups gluten-free all-purpose baking flour
1-teaspoon baking soda
1/4 teaspoon salt
1/2 cup soymilk
2 cups mashed ripe bananas (4-5 medium)
3/4 cup sugar
1/4 cup brown sugar
1/2 cup unsweetened applesauce
1/3 cup canola oil
1/2 tsp. cinnamon
1-teaspoon vanilla extract
2 T Maple Syrup
First, mix all dry ingredients in a mixing bowl, set aside.

Combine wet ingredients, mix well and add to dry ingredients.

Place dough in two 8x4 inch loaf pans and bake at 350 degrees for approximately 45 minutes. Loafs tend to be a bit crumbly so allow to cool for several minutes before removing from loaf pans. Your friends will never know this is a gluten free vegan recipe!

Vegan Gluten Free Chocolate Chip Cookies

As you know, most chocolate chips are not on the vegan approved grocery list so you may have despaired ever smelling the chocolate goodness that is the chocolate chip cookie. Rest assured there is a gluten free vegan alternative.

1/2 C Tapioca Starch
1/2 C brown rice flour
1/2 C sorghum flour
1/2 C potato starch
1/2 C Granulated sugar
1/2 teaspoon xanthan gum
1/2 teaspoon baking soda
1/2 teaspoon salt
1/2 C grape seed oil
3/4 C pure maple syrup
2 teaspoons vanilla
1/2-3/4 cup vegan chocolate chips

Mix together dry ingredients in a medium mixing bowl. Next stir in vanilla, oil and maple syrup. You can mix ingredients by hand or use a mechanical mixer on a medium setting. Mixture will be slightly thin but add in chocolate chips and allow to stand for about 10 minutes.

It will thicken up.

Drop cookie dough on prepared baking sheets by the tablespoon and bake for around 10 minutes. Cookies should look a bit doughy and underdone. Allow to cool on the baking sheet for a few minutes, (cookies will continue to cook for a bit after coming out of the oven.)

Soups

Sometimes nothing satisfies like a warm bowl of tasty soup. If you are tired of trying to find a good gluten free vegan soup from the canned varieties in your local store, here are a few homemade soups to add to your recipe box.

Gluten Free Vegan Tomato Soup

Are you feeling a bit under the weather? Perhaps you just want something that is filling but light on the stomach at the same time. Gluten free vegan tomato soup sounds like the perfect solution.

2 cans Stewed Tomatoes
1 large carrot.
1 large turnip.
1 large onion.
2 1/4 cups of water.
3 ounces vegan butter.
1-tablespoon sago.
2 teaspoons salt.

1 tsp. dried tarragon
1-tablespoon lemon juice
Pepper to taste

Dice onion, carrot, and turnip. In a medium saucepan heat half vegan, butter sauté gently. Add pepper, salt and water to mix and boil gently. Once vegetables are quite tender pour in stewed tomatoes, salt to taste and other half of vegan butter. Simmer all ingredients together with tarragon, lemon juice and pepper for approximately 60 minutes or until vegetables are thoroughly cooked. Allow mixture to cool slightly then puree until smooth and enjoy.

Hearty Mexican Soup

Here is a favorite that is a little heartier than your traditional soup!

1 can chili beans
1 can pinto beans
½ C onion- finely chopped
1 can stewed tomatoes (diced works as well)
2 tsp. ground cumin
1 tsp. chili powder
1 tsp. paprika
Garlic powder to taste
1 ½ C water

Bring all ingredients to a boil in a medium saucepan. Reduce heat and simmer for 15-20 minutes. Serve with your favorite gluten free vegan chips, sour cream and vegan cheese!

Reduce water to increase consistency and this makes a great filler for corn tortilla. One recipe that doubles as two meals.

Potato, Squash and Apple Soup

You might be a little ambiguous about adding apples to a vegetable soup recipe, but give it a chance. This might just become your favorite cold weather concoction.

1/2 butternut squash
1 medium red potatoes
2 or more garlic cloves- minced
1 green apples, peeled and chopped
Salt and pepper to taste
1-2 sprigs of fresh thyme (1/2 tsp. of dried can be substituted)
Olive oil
2 cups of vegetable stock

Prepare squash and potatoes. Peel, de-seed squash and cut both into bite-sized cubes. Next peel, core and quarter green apple. Set aside.

Sauté minced garlic with olive oil in a medium sized stockpot. Cook until golden. Add vegetables and apple to your sautéed garlic and cook for a few minutes. (2-5) Next add vegetable stock, reduce heat and allow soup to simmer until potatoes and squash are fork tender.

French Cabbage Soup

Who said vegan and gluten free recipes had to be all-American? Take the French cabbage soup out for a test drive today!

3 carrots
1 turnip
1 leek
2 sticks celery
1/2 cabbage
1 bay leaf
2 whole cloves
5 peppercorns
12 C. water.

Peel and dice carrots and turnips, dice celery, slice the leek and shred the 1/2 head of cabbage.

Place all ingredients together in a large stockpot. Bring water and vegetables to a boil and then reduce heat. Allow soup to simmer on low for 2-3 hours. At the end of the day, you have a delicious, healthy soup.

Raw Foods, Seasonal Favorites and Drinks

You might think adding another diet category to a gluten free vegan lifestyle would be unnecessarily difficult, but when that category is raw food, it actually makes a lot of sense. Gluten free and vegan fit very nicely with a raw food diet, and gives you a few more recipe alternatives.

Pineapple Banana Drink

1 C fresh banana
1 C fresh pineapple
2 C spinach
1/2 C water
2-3 regular ice cubes

Place all ingredients in a blender and process on high speeds until contents are smooth. You can ditch the ice by using frozen produce instead. You should know this drink will be quite green, thanks to the spinach!

Bacon- Sort Of!

Do you ever get a hankering for some good old-fashioned bacon? What if you could achieve the flavor and texture without betraying your vegan lifestyle? Enter eggplant bacon!

1 lb. eggplant
4 TBS gluten free soy sauce
1 tsp. liquid smoke

Create a marinade from the gluten free soy sauce and liquid smoke, set aside. Cut your eggplant in to small strips, about 1/8 inch to be exact. Place eggplant strips in marinade, making sure each piece is covered well. Allow vegetable to soak for at least a couple of hours.

At this point you have a couple of alternatives, you can use a dehydrator set on 116 for approximately 12 hours or bake your eggplant bacon. Pre-heat oven to 425 degrees and bake for 8-10 minutes turning once and baking for another 2-4 minutes. The result is a bacon alternative that you can eat alone or as a topping for your favorite dish. (Perhaps a gluten free vegan baked potato?)

"Eggnog"

Have you always enjoyed the holidays and in particular eggnog? You will probably be hard pressed to find a good tasting vegan eggnog, so why not make your own?

1/2 cup cashews
1/2 cup macadamia nuts
2 cups water
Sea salt to taste
6 tbs. agave nectar
Pinch of nutmeg

In your trusty blender process, all ingredients until they are relatively smooth. Remove any small particles of nuts by running your mixture through a cheesecloth or something similar. Serve slightly chilled and enjoy.

Vegan Cocoa

Another seasonal favorite that many hate to mark off their list is hot chocolate or cocoa. Good news, you do not have to!

1 C almond milk
1 1/2 T cocoa powder (unsweetened of course)
2 tsp. sugar

In a small saucepan, cook almond milk until it is steaming hot, but not boiling. Stir in sugar and cocoa mix, add a stick of cinnamon on the side and you are ready to settle in on any chilly evening.

Holiday Favorite Pumpkin Pie

1 16 oz. can pumpkin

½ C granulated sugar

¼ C brown sugar

1 C soy milk (almond is good too)

1 tsp. vanilla

¼ tsp. nutmeg

¼ tsp. allspice

½ tsp. cinnamon

1 gluten free pie crust (purchased or made from recipe above)

Blend all ingredients in a medium mixing bowl with an electric hand mixer on low speeds. Mix for 3-4 minutes. Pour mixture into gluten free vegan pie shells, insert into 425-degree oven for 15 minutes. Turn down oven to 350 degrees and bake for about 45 minutes. Allow dish to cool before consuming.

Gluten Free Vegan Staples for the Pantry

Now that you have made the decision to change your life, what do you need to do first? If you have always consumed a traditional diet, you may want to start slowly by choosing a few items to replace as you learn new recipes. You have several alternative items to work with, which means it could get expensive quickly. Choose one or two from each category to begin your transition to a healthier lifestyle.

- Oils
- Extra virgin olive oil
- Saffron Oil
- Coconut oil
- Sunflower oil
- Beans
- Pinto
- Navy
- Kidney
- Black-eyed Peas
- (pretty much any dried bean is good for a gluten free vegan diet)

- Whole Grain Flour
- Cornmeal
- Quinoa
- Spelt
- Rice flour
- Herbs and Spices

This is another category where pretty much anything goes, however two come to mind as particularly useful.

Italian Seasoning
Curry powder

Finally-

Fruits, vegetables and rice tend to be fantastic starter foods for a gluten free vegan diet. There are so many dishes you can create with these ingredients and some imagination!

Health Concerns of a Vegan Gluten Free Diet

The general consensus for the health of a gluten free vegan diet is that it is good, provided you are willing to supplement your diet to make up for a few key vitamins and minerals that will be lacking. By excluding both dairy and meat products from your diet you lose several key minerals and vitamins. If you want to be successful and healthy with this type of restrictive diet, here are a few of the supplements you will need to consume.

Vitamin B-12

Vitamin B-12 is very important to the healthy function of the human body. B-12 is necessary for the production of red blood cells, which carry much needed oxygen throughout the body. Deficiencies in this vitamin can lead to lethargy and weakness.

Foods rich in B-12 include:
Beef liver
Clams
Rainbow trout

Eggs
Chicken breast

You cannot get enough vitamin B-12 from your diet when you follow a gluten free vegan lifestyle. Thankfully, there are supplements on the market to help you make up for the short fall in your daily diet.

Iron

Another building block of blood is iron, which is typically found in adequate levels if you eat a varied diet. Vegans and vegetarians, however, have such a limited diet it is difficult to get adequate amounts from food alone since the richest sources are items such as:

Calf liver
Cooked oysters
Cuttlefish
Octopus
Beef heart
Various organ meats

You will probably here a lot of people tout the iron levels of soybeans, lentils, spinach and various other vegetables but you should know these are two different types of iron. Meat based iron is known as Heme-iron while plant based is non-heme. The major difference in the two is absorption rates, heme iron absorbs much more readily than non-heme varieties. Therefore, if you are vegan or vegetarian you should make it a point to consume more iron rich vegetables such as kale, broccoli and legumes (beans).

Omega-3 Fatty Acids

The loss of eggs and fish from your diet leave you at risk for omega-3 deficiencies. Cold water fish such as sardines and mackerel are two of the best sources of this essential nutrient. However, walnuts, flaxseed oil, soybeans and canola oil are great sources as well. Many people opt for fish oil capsules as a supplement, but that may not sit well with your vegan lifestyle.

Calcium

Your bones and teeth depend on adequate calcium, without it, you could face tooth loss and early onset osteoporosis or worse. Most people do not realize that calcium deficiency can leave you vulnerable to hypertension, abnormal heartbeat and in severe cases convulsions!

Calcium also plays a major role in many other functions of the human body such as hormone secretion, nerve transmission, muscle stimulation and so much more. Calcium deficiency can lead to brittle nails; hair loss, heart arrhythmia, anxiety and severe irritation just to name a few.

Since milk, cheese and fish are off the menu it is important that you consume a diet high in plant-based calcium and take vitamin D supplements. Vitamin D is necessary for calcium absorption and is another vitamin taken off the menu with the vegan gluten free diet.

Gluten Free Concerns

In most cases there are no real risks with a gluten free diet, in fact the human body does not absorb gluten but passes it through the digestive system. The biggest concern with this type of limiting diet is nutrition. As with a vegan diet, there are a few essential vitamins and minerals you will be missing out on, and since many people replace, breads with higher calorie nuts you could theoretically gain weight on a gluten free diet.

If you feel you may have a gluten sensitivity or celiac

disease it is important that you talk to your medical professional. Ask him or her to perform the necessary blood test to confirm your suspicions, before you begin a specialized diet. Celiac disease symptoms are relatively common and similar to several other ailments, so you may have to ask for the test specifically as many doctors do not think to perform it as a routine test.

Gluten Free Vegan Conclusion

Is it possible to lead a gluten free vegan life? A few years ago, the outlook would have been grim but thanks to the wide variety of gluten free and vegan friendly products on the market today it has never been easier. More importantly, it is now possible to follow this type of diet and still be able to consume great tasting dishes. There are a few concerns and questions that come up when considering a radical change, here are a few of the most common.

Vegan FAQ's

Is a vegan diet healthy?

According to the American Dietetic Association, there is no reason a vegetarian or vegan diet cannot provide a nutritional alternative. That being said, your diet needs to be well planned so that all your essential vitamins, minerals and fatty acids are accounted for, as mentioned above.

How difficult is it to go vegan?

Depending on how rigidly you plan to adhere to the vegan principles, it can be very difficult at first. The key to making this type of transition is to start slowly, making small changes. Any step toward an animal friendly existence is a good one.

Is a vegan diet expensive?

Again, this depends a lot on your approach. Purchasing the majority of your diet in the form of pre-packaged vegan alternatives can get quite expensive. However, if you compare the cost of vegetables, beans and other staple vegan items with the rising costs of meat you may find the vegan diet is quite a bit cheaper.

Gluten Free FAQ's

What foods can I eat?

It is actually easier to discuss what you should avoid. Any foods that contain wheat, rye and barley are out of the question. The key is to learn which items on an ingredient list are derived from one of the above. For example malt, triticale and malt vinegar are all derived from items on the banned list.

Why are oats such a big deal?

Pure oats are gluten free and perfectly acceptable on a gluten free diet. However, until recently commercially packaged oats were often exposed to cross contamination from wheat, rye or barley. Read your labels carefully, particularly if you are a celiac sufferer.

Is celiac disease really that bad?

Over time and left untreated celiac disease can cause a variety of health problems. Since the villi in the intestine are continually destroyed it becomes harder and harder for the body to get the nutrition it needs. This can lead to brittle bones, skin conditions, anemia and other ailments.

Should you start a gluten free vegan diet today? Whether you suffer celiac disease or simply want a diet plan that puts you on the right track to losing weight and feeling better this could be the answer for you.

Create a plan for putting this diet in place, after all if you have always lived a traditional lifestyle it can be quite a shock to just empty the pantry and refrigerator and start on what may seem like a foreign diet.

Baby Steps

In the beginning, the easiest transition will be away from meat products. Slowly begin phasing out your favorite meat dishes for healthier vegetarian options. This is a good time to begin experimenting with tofu and different ways to create mock meat dishes. Silken tofu is a good option and can be processed to resemble ground beef for Italian dishes.

CAUTION: If you do opt for vegan meat alternatives found in the grocery store you should read the labels carefully. Many of these products contain wheat, rye or barley and are not appropriate for a gluten free diet.

Next, you could switch your whole, two percent or skim milk for a soy or nut milk alternative. There are several commercially produced non-dairy milks on the shelves today thanks to the number of people who are lactose intolerant. Do not be afraid to try different brands and types of milk until you find one that suits your taste buds.

Keep it Simple

Vegan and gluten free recipes are very easy to find, however not all of them are simple. When you are first starting out keep it simple. Complicated recipes can result in at best a tasteless dish and at worst something, you would not feed your dog! This could derail your entire plan for a gluten free vegan diet, so opt for easy to make recipes that do not contain a large number of bizarre ingredients or spices.

Substitute

Do you have some favorite recipes you would really hate to give up on? Work on making vegan and gluten free substitutions. While this might seem like a daunting task at first, you will soon discover which binding agents work best in each type of recipe and which vegetables can be substituted for meat or gluten based products.

NOTE: This task is not for the faint at heart or those who are easily discouraged. Be prepared to throw away and laugh at some of your more epic failures. It is through this process you will grow and become a more knowledgeable cook and successful vegan.

Gluten Free Vegan -- In Summary

A gluten free vegan diet may not sound like the easiest path in the world to take, but when your health is on the line, it is definitely worth the trouble. Plan your progress, choose nutrient high foods and take the appropriate supplements when necessary. Talk to your medical professional about monitoring for things like calcium, B-12, iron and magnesium.

Lightning Source UK Ltd.
Milton Keynes UK
UKOW01f1235060218
317442UK00009B/377/P